UNDERSTANDING NORDIC WALKING FOR BEGINNERS

Advance Guide To Unlock The Secrets Of Nordic Walking, Discover The Joy, Health Benefits, And Essential Techniques Of This Invigorating Outdoor Exercise

KIERAN RAJESH

CHAPTER 1
INTRODUCTION TO NORDIC WALKING

Nordic Walking, an increasingly popular fitness activity on a global scale, is a full-body workout that utilizes poles that have been specifically intended for this purpose. By integrating components of walking and cross-country skiing, this type of physical activity concurrently targets the upper body, abdominal muscles, and lower limbs. Nordic Walking originated in Finland during the 1930s when cross-country skiers were actively seeking methods to sustain their physical endurance throughout the off-season. After its inception, it has transformed, becoming a multipurpose and readily available mode of physical activity that is appropriate for individuals across all age groups and levels of fitness. This introductory section examines the historical evolution of Nordic Walking and its multifarious advantages, delving into its definition and origins.

The Origins and Definition

Nordic walking is a physically demanding activity characterized by the use of poles that are specifically engineered for walking, resembling those employed in cross-country skiing. By requiring the use of the upper extremities, the activity stimulates the entire body, setting it apart from conventional strolling. The practice of Nordic Walking originated in Finland during the early 20th century. In the beginning, this activity was designed to provide cross-country skiers with a means to maintain cardiovascular fitness, muscle, and endurance during the snow-free months. The utilization of poles as a means to augment the walking experience progressively garnered attention, developing into a discernible and extensively implemented mode of physical activity.

The development of Nordic Walking

The progression of Nordic Walking has been characterized by a shift from a specialized form of training intended for athletes to a widely recognized fitness activity that is available to a wider demographic. During the early years, cross-country skiers seeking a way to maintain fitness outside of the skiing season were the primary target audience. The momentum of its evolution increased during the 1990s when fitness professionals and Nordic walking enthusiasts began to acknowledge its capacity to enhance general health and well-being. As a result, non-athletes were provided with apparatus, training programs, and specialized techniques that catered to their requirements. As the popularity of Nordic Walking has increased as a fitness and recreational activity, an expanding body of scientific research has confirmed its effectiveness in enhancing muscular strength, cardiovascular fitness, and flexibility.

The advantages of Nordic walking

The numerous mental, physical, and social advantages of Nordic walking contribute to its immense popularity. Physically speaking, the utilization of upper body muscles during this activity leads to a more holistic exercise in comparison to conventional walking.

By distributing the load across the entire body, the use of poles reduces joint stress and encourages improved posture. As a result, Nordic Walking is appropriate for people of all fitness levels and physical conditions. Extensive research has established the cardiovascular advantages of Nordic Walking, including enhanced endurance, improved cardiac health, and increased oxygen consumption. Furthermore, research has demonstrated that engaging in this activity can aid in the prevention of chronic ailments, including diabetes and hypertension, as well as aid in weight management.

The positive effects of Nordic walking on mental health are also significant. The activity's rhythmic and repetitive characteristics induce a state of relaxation, aiding in the reduction of tension and mental unwinding. Nordic Walking, being an external activity, facilitates individuals' connection with nature, thereby promoting a sense of tranquillity and alleviating symptoms associated with anxiety and depression. Additionally, the communal nature of Nordic Walking, which is frequently undertaken in organizations or groups, promotes a feeling of camaraderie and assistance. The inclusion of this social aspect enhances motivation, compliance with the activity, and overall psychological welfare.

To summarise, Nordic walking has transformed a specialized training technique favoured by athletes into a widely recognized fitness activity. In contrast to conventional strolling, its definition is predicated on the utilization of poles that have been specifically engineered for this purpose. Nordic Walking's versatility and inclusiveness are underscored by its origins in Finland and subsequent global evolution. The manifold advantages, which encompass improved physical fitness, psychological equilibrium, and social engagement, emphasize the diverse allure of this activity and establish it as a valuable supplement to the collection of physical pursuits for those in pursuit of a comprehensive approach to well-being and physical fitness.

CHAPTER 2
EQUIPMENT AND GEAR OF THE NECESSARY

Nordic walking, an exercise regimen that integrates strolling with the utilization of purpose-built poles, requires the application of indispensable gear and equipment to optimize its advantages and guarantee a secure and pleasurable encounter. The Nordic walking poles are essential components of the Nordic walking apparatus, functioning as the principal implements to activate the upper body throughout the exercise routine. In contrast to conventional hiking or trekking poles, these poles are constructed with particular attention to detail to support the distinctive motions associated with Nordic walking. Consideration must be given to the length, material, and grip of these poles when choosing the appropriate combination for a given individual's requirements.

<u>Walking Nordic poles:</u>

The utilization of Nordic walking poles is crucial to the exercise's efficacy, as they function as arm extensions that stimulate the muscles of the upper body. Aluminum or carbon fiber are common lightweight materials used to construct these poles to facilitate portability and usability. The efficiency of the walking technique and the level of commitment of the upper body musculature are both significantly influenced by the length of the poles. Poles of appropriate dimensions facilitate an organic arm oscillation and encourage an erect posture, thereby mitigating joint strain.

The handles, frequently featuring wrist straps, facilitate the efficient transmission of force through the poles and offer a secure hold. Individuals must comprehend the intricacies of Nordic walking pole design to select the apparatus that is most appropriate for their individual preferences and level of physical fitness.

<u>Selecting Appropriate Footwear:</u>

The selection of footwear has a substantial impact on the overall efficacy and experience of Nordic walking. In contrast to conventional running or walking shoes, Nordic walking shoes are engineered to deliver the precise stability, support, and flexibility required for the associated movements.

To promote comfort during extended treks while adhering to the required ground contact for stability, the footwear ought to provide an equilibrium between responsiveness and cushioning. Arch support, heel-to-toe drop, and overall fit are elements that participants should take into account to mitigate discomfort and minimize the likelihood of sustaining injuries. Furthermore, the outsole of Nordic walking shoes must offer sufficient traction on a diverse range of surfaces, such as gravel, pavement, and the undulating terrains that are frequently encountered throughout Nordic walking sessions.

<u>Sufficient Garments for Nordic Walking:</u>

The careful consideration of appropriate attire is critical for Nordic walkers to ensure both comfort and optimal performance, given the unpredictable weather conditions and physical demands associated with the activity.

The utilization of moisture-wicking and lightweight fabrics is critical for the regulation of body temperature and the facilitation of perspiration. By utilizing layering, individuals can modify their attire in response to changes in temperature and physical activity. Base and mid-layers aid in temperature regulation, whereas an outer layer that is breathable and weather-resistant offers protection from rain and wind. A tailored fit on apparel prevents chafing and facilitates a complete range of motion. Particular emphasis should be placed on accessories such as sunglasses, mittens, and hats, as they provide supplementary protection and augment the overall comfort of Nordic walkers across various weather conditions.

<u>Additional Accessories to Improve Performance:</u>

In addition to clothing, footwear, and poles, a variety of accessories can improve the efficacy and enjoyment of Nordic walking. A suitable carrying system for the Nordic walking poles is an essential accessory, as it enables users to secure the poles when not in use. This functionality proves to be especially beneficial when taking pauses or switching between walking and other pursuits. Hydration systems, including hydration packs and water bottles, are indispensable for optimal performance maintenance, particularly during longer Nordic walking excursions. Fitness sensors and heart rate monitors provide vital information for monitoring progress and optimizing training intensity. Gaiters and thermal socks may be required in colder climates to keep feet toasty and dry. Gaining an understanding of the function of these accessories and integrating them into the Nordic walking regimen enhances the overall experience by promoting physical health and overall activity satisfaction.

CHAPTER 3
FORM AND APPROPRIATE METHODOLOGY

To fully benefit from the dynamic and total-body nature of Nordic walking, appropriate technique and form knowledge are essential. The foundation of Nordic walking consists of traversing with ski pole-like poles that have been specially designed. Nordic walking requires precise form and technique to be an effective exercise that reduces the risk of injury.

When establishing the correct form and technique for Nordic walking, it is critical to place significant emphasis on maintaining a straight posture. Sustaining an erect alignment accompanied by a modest forward lean effectively utilizes the core muscles and enhances overall stability.

Shoulders should be relaxed and the vertebrae straight to facilitate a natural arm swing. Adequate body alignment guarantees the even distribution of forces generated during every stride, thereby averting excessive strain on particular joints.

In addition, weight distribution is a critical component of the Nordic walking technique.

A seamless transition of weight from one foot to the other should occur during each stride to promote a rhythmic and fluent motion.

This weight transfer promotes strength and endurance by engaging the lower body muscles, including the quadriceps, hamstrings, and glutes. The maintenance of regulated weight distribution is critical for the prevention of muscle imbalances and the mitigation of overuse injuries.

3.1 Fundamental Nordic Walking Position:

The fundamental Nordic walking posture serves as the cornerstone of the entire technique. This particular position entails a deliberate alignment of the torso, limbs, and feet to maximize the effectiveness of the locomotion process. By positioning the feet hip-width apart, one can establish a stable foundation. To ensure a cushioned landing and to dissipate shock, the knees are bent slightly with each step. Additionally, this knee flexion facilitates leg muscle engagement throughout the walking cycle.

The placement of the arms is a fundamental component of the Nordic walking posture.

The reciprocal motion of the arms resembles the arm swing that naturally transpires during ordinary strolling. By positioning the poles behind the body and angling them slightly in the backward direction, the walker is propelled forward through a push-off motion. A neutral position should be maintained with the wrists while preserving a firm but relaxed grip on the poles. Ensuring accurate arm alignment facilitates the transfer of maximum power from the upper body to the legs, thereby augmenting the overall efficacy of the walking technique.

In addition, it is beneficial to perform a minor rotation of the torso during each stride to stimulate the core muscles. By incorporating this rotational motion, not only is stability enhanced, but the engagement of the abdominal muscles is also optimized. When performed accurately, the fundamental Nordic walking stance incorporates the complete body into the motion of walking, thereby converting an ordinary stroll into a comprehensive exercise regimen for the entire body.

3.2 Swing of the Arm and Pole Position:

The arm motion and pole placement are essential elements of Nordic walking that substantially enhance its efficacy as a full-body exercise. Effective coordination between arm movement and pole placement improves balance and stability while increasing the engagement of upper body muscles.

It is imperative to comprehend the intricacies of arm motion and pole placement to attain ideal outcomes and mitigate the risk of potential injuries.

Similar to conventional strolling, Nordic walking involves an arm swing that is intensified to accommodate the use of poles. Each step causes the arms to advance, resulting in the poles being positioned behind the body at a minor outward angle. Complementing the efforts of the lower body, this motion engages the triceps, biceps, and shoulder muscles, thereby providing an upper-body exercise.

By maintaining a fluid and controlled arm swing, one should prevent the shoulders and forearms from experiencing undue tension.

Pole placement must be optimized to fully benefit from Nordic walking. Each stride should involve planting the poles diagonally behind the body, extending them backward. By adopting this stance, the walker can generate a push-off motion that advances it, thereby generating momentum and elevating the cardiovascular requirements of the activity. Additionally, it is imperative to consider the length of the poles, as adjusting them will guarantee a comfortable and effective reach while mitigating superfluous strain on the arms and shoulders.

Additionally, the intensity of Nordic walking is influenced by the angle at which the poles are elevated. An elongated pole angle enhances cardiovascular and endurance advantages, whereas a marginally advanced pole angle stimulates upper-body muscle engagement. It is critical to comprehend the correlation between pole placement and arm motion to customize the exercise regimen to suit individual fitness objectives and guarantee an equitable dispersion of exertion between the lower and upper extremities.

3.3 Length of Stride and Cadence:

The overall effectiveness of Nordic walking is considerably impacted by stride length and cadence, which are fundamental components of the exercise. Attaining an optimal equilibrium between stride length and cadence not only amplifies the cardiovascular advantages but also promotes appropriate muscle activation and joint well-being. A comprehensive comprehension of the principles underlying stride length and cadence is of the utmost importance for those who wish to maximize their Nordic walking experience.

The stride duration in Nordic walking should be deliberate and under control. Engaging in excessive striding or prolonged walking can result in unwarranted stress on the joints, specifically the knees. In contrast, exercising with inadequate stride length could restrict leg muscle engagement and diminish the overall efficacy of the routine. Maintaining proper form while striking a balance between a comfortable gait length and energy transfer facilitates the effective exchange of force and reduces the likelihood of physical harm.

In Nordic walking, cadence, or the number of strides performed per minute, is an additional crucial factor. It is generally advised to maintain a moderate cadence to strike a balance between cardiovascular exertion and muscle involvement. While there may be some variation in the optimal cadence between individuals, striving for a steady and rhythmic pace facilitates consistent cardiovascular exercise while reducing the likelihood of fatigue. Additionally, synchronizing arm swing, pole positioning, and overall body movement with cadence facilitates the formation of a streamlined and harmonious walking pattern.

In addition, it is critical to adapt stride length and cadence in Nordic walking in response to the terrain. Alterations to maintain equilibrium and control may be necessary on ascending or descending slopes. In ascending terrain, one can enhance their ability to conquer the incline by reducing their stride length and increasing their cadence. On the contrary, when traversing downhill segments, keeping your stride slightly longer while maintaining a controlled cadence helps to preserve your stability and prevents undue strain on your joints.

3.4 Frequent Errors and Methods for Preventing Them:

Although Nordic walking provides a multitude of advantages when executed properly, there are prevalent errors that individuals may unintentionally commit, which can result in diminished efficacy and potential hazards of injury. Acknowledging these errors and comprehending the means to circumvent them is critical in fostering a secure and effective Nordic walking encounter.

A prevalent error is inadequate pole placement, in which participants position the poles at an incorrect angle or too far in front of their bodies. This phenomenon not only reduces the activation of the upper body muscles but also interferes with the organic rhythm of walking. To mitigate this issue, individuals who engage in walking should concentrate on positioning the poles diagonally behind the body, guaranteeing that the action coincides with the arm movement that occurs naturally.

Arm motion inconsistency is an additional common error observed in Nordic walking. Certain individuals may engage in excessive arm swinging, which can result in shoulder tension; conversely, others may utilize their arms insufficiently, which can diminish the overall upper body workout. By coordinating the placement of the pole with a balanced and controlled arm swing, it is possible to effectively engage the muscles in the back, shoulders, and arms while minimizing superfluous strain.

Mistaken posture has the potential to undermine the advantages associated with Nordic strolling. Excessive forward leaning or slouching can potentially result in back discomfort and diminished activation of the core muscles. It is essential to sustain an upright posture with a slight forward lean to optimize the efficacy of the walking motion and distribute forces uniformly throughout the body.

Overstriding, which involves taking steps that are too lengthy, is a prevalent mistake that can heighten the likelihood of experiencing joint strain and fatigue. It is advised that individuals maintain a deliberate and regulated gait length, preventing the use of excessive steps that could potentially harm joint health. The use of short, rapid movements accompanied by a moderate cadence enhances the effectiveness and sustainability of the Nordic walking technique.

Finally, it is a critical error to disregard the significance of warm-up and cool-down procedures, as doing so can compromise the overall safety and efficacy of Nordic walking. By warming up the muscles before commencing the exercise and integrating a progressive cool-down at its conclusion, one can effectively mitigate the risk of injuries, enhance flexibility, and facilitate muscle recovery.

Nordic walking is an adaptable and efficacious exercise regimen that targets the muscles of the upper and lower body, thereby providing an extensive array of health advantages. For optimal stride length and cadence, as well as mastery of the fundamental Nordic walking posture, arm swing, and pole placement, proper technique and form are crucial. By doing so, one can fully benefit from this activity. Acquiring knowledge regarding prevalent errors and strategies to circumvent them further guarantees a secure and pleasurable Nordic walking encounter. By adopting the principles delineated in each concept, individuals have the potential to augment their competence in Nordic walking, resulting in enhanced physical fitness, cardiovascular health, and general welfare.

CHAPTER 4
FITNESS AND HEALTH BENEFITS

<u>Cardiovascular Advantages:</u>

Nordic walking, an exercise regimen that integrates the utilization of purpose-engineered poles, provides an extensive array of cardiovascular advantages. By involving the entire body, this low-impact exercise promotes cardiovascular health. In conjunction with the use of walking poles, the rhythmic arm and limb movements increase heart rate and stimulate blood circulation. Engaging in this aerobic exercise, which is comparable to jogging or brisk strolling, enhances cardiovascular endurance. Research has indicated that engaging in Nordic walking can result in elevated cardiac output and improved oxygen consumption, which in turn fortifies the heart and diminishes the likelihood of developing cardiovascular ailments. Additionally, compared to conventional walking, the utilization of both upper and lower body muscle groups is involved, which contributes to a more comprehensive cardiovascular exercise.

Engagement of Muscles and Toning:

A distinguishing characteristic of Nordic Walking is its capacity to simultaneously engage multiple muscle groups.

The incorporation of walking poles into the walking motion stimulates the upper back, shoulders, and arm muscles, resulting in a synchronized interaction with the lower body muscles. The comprehensive involvement of all muscles in this process results in enhanced muscular tone and endurance. In addition to engaging the main muscle groups, Nordic walking also strengthens the stabilizing muscles, which improves balance and coordination.

The resistance introduced by the poles' constant push-and-pull motion enhances the exercise and promotes the development of muscular strength. Consequently, those who engage in Nordic Walking demonstrate improved muscular toning, specifically in the abdominal region, upper body, and lower extremities, culminating in a physique that is more harmonious and sculpted.

Management of Body Weight via Nordic Walking:

Individuals in search of a productive method to regulate their body weight will find Nordic Walking to be an advantageous exercise regimen. In comparison to conventional pacing, the combination of cardiovascular and muscular engagement results in a greater expenditure of calories. In conjunction with a well-balanced diet, this increased caloric expenditure promotes weight management and aids in the process of weight reduction. The energy expenditure is increased during Nordic walking due to its capacity to engage muscles in both the upper and lower body, rendering it a more effective activity for burning calories. In addition, the increased metabolic rate after physical activity, referred to as excess post-exercise oxygen consumption (EPOC), contributes to the maintenance of a healthy weight by encouraging sustained calorie expenditure following the exertion. Nordic walking is therefore an effective and environmentally friendly option for those who wish to attain and sustain a healthy body weight.

<u>The Effects on Joint Health:</u>

Nordic walking distinguishes itself as a low-impact, joint-friendly form of exercise, rendering it an appealing choice for individuals who have concerns related to the joints. By distributing the impact of each stride across the upper and lower body, walking poles alleviate stress on joints such as the knees and hips. As a result, Nordic Walking is feasible for a wider range of individuals, including those who suffer from arthritis or joint discomfort. Research has indicated that engaging in Nordic walking may enhance joint flexibility and range of motion, thereby potentially mitigating symptoms that are commonly associated with specific joint disorders. The activity's controlled and supportive characteristics render it a highly suitable option for individuals seeking to incorporate consistent physical activity into their routine without aggravating joint pain. In general, the beneficial effects of Nordic Walking on joint health establish it as a worthwhile choice for those in search of fitness activities that are gentle on the joints.

Nordic walking is a multifaceted form of physical activity that presents an extensive array of health advantages. Due to its notable cardiovascular benefits, which include improved endurance and decreased risk of cardiovascular complications, this exercise is deemed efficacious in fostering cardiac well-being. By stimulating multiple muscle groups, which results in enhanced balance and tone, this form of exercise expands the scope of muscular fitness beyond conventional strolling. Additionally, its capacity for weight management and its favourable impact on joints render Nordic Walking a flexible and approachable option for people with diverse health conditions and levels of physical fitness. With the increasing pursuit of holistic approaches to health and well-being, Nordic Walking emerges as a compelling alternative that effectively tackles health and fitness considerations.

CHAPTER 5
ADAPTING NORDIC WALKING TO VARIOUS FITNESS LEVELS

Nordic walking is an adaptable form of physical activity that accommodates participants of different fitness levels. A comprehensive guide is imperative for novices to establish the groundwork for a prosperous

Nordic walking expedition. It is imperative to acquaint novice practitioners with the foundational techniques, apparatus, and biomechanics associated with this extraordinary Endeavor. A proper gait length, handgrip, and posture are critical elements that novices must master to prevent injuries and maximize the benefits of Nordic walking. It is crucial to commence with fewer sessions and progressively escalate the duration and intensity as one develops expertise. Furthermore, the integration of warm-up and cool-down protocols specifically designed for Nordic walking can augment the exercise's overall efficacy while mitigating the potential for muscular strain.

Sophisticated Methods for Experienced Walkers

As individuals advance in their Nordic walking endeavours, they might be inclined to investigate more sophisticated techniques to push the boundaries of their physical capabilities and enrich the overall experience. Nordic walking progression entails the enhancement of foundational techniques and the integration of more dynamic motions. Expert pedestrians may wish to concentrate on improving their gait, acquiring more intricate pole manoeuvres, and integrating hill climbs or interval training into their regimen. Achieving proficiency in utilizing terrain variations, honing arm movements, and synchronizing pole placements are all fundamental elements of advanced Nordic walking. Involvement in extended and more rigorous Nordic walking sessions necessitates knowledge of appropriate cadence and strategies for developing endurance. Additionally, advanced users can derive advantages from employing specialized Nordic walking poles that are engineered to tackle particular terrain obstacles.

The Nordic Walk for the Elderly

Nordic walking exhibits tremendous promise as a low-impact, senior-friendly form of exercise, imparting a multitude of health advantages while preventing undue stress on the joints. Seniors must adopt a modified Nordic walking regimen to accommodate their specific requirements and potential physical constraints. Promoting balance, coordination, and cardiovascular health ought to be the primary focus. Adapting the walking sessions to a more moderate tempo and integrating light stretching exercises can effectively address the unique needs of the senior population. Furthermore, it is critical to prioritize the selection of suitable Nordic walking poles that possess adjustable lengths and ergonomic attributes to guarantee senior citizens' comfort and stability throughout their sessions.

This particular mode of physical activity not only promotes physical health but also facilitates social interaction, thus constituting a comprehensive pursuit for older adults.

Nordic walking integration into cross-training

Nordic walking functions as a harmonious incorporation into cross-training regimens, providing a comprehensive approach to overall physical fitness. Cross-training is a method that combines a variety of exercises to strengthen and condition across multiple muscle groups. By incorporating Nordic walking into a cross-training regimen, one can supplement other forms of exercise, such as strength training, cycling, or swimming, with full-body exertion. Nordic walking is an optimal form of cross-training due to its distinctive characteristic of appealing to both the upper and lower body muscles. Gaining an understanding of the interplay between Nordic walking and other forms of exercise enables individuals to develop a comprehensive fitness regimen that targets diverse facets of fitness. Furthermore, its versatility renders Nordic walking an appropriate form of exercise for individuals seeking to achieve particular fitness objectives, such as weight reduction, muscle development, or cardiovascular well-being.

Nordic walking presents a flexible and all-encompassing mode of physical activity that can be adapted to accommodate individuals with varying degrees of fitness. The foundation for novices is established in an exhaustive beginners' guide, which emphasizes correct techniques and gradual progression. Sophisticated walkers are accommodated by advanced techniques, which incorporate dynamic movements and variations in terrain. Nordic walking is considered appropriate for senior citizens due to its low-impact characteristics and ability to adjust to account for age-related factors. Incorporating Nordic walking into cross-training regimens complements other forms of exercise and provides a full-body routine, thereby enhancing overall fitness. Comprehending these principles enables individuals to experience the multifarious advantages of Nordic walking, thereby establishing it as a valuable supplement to a comprehensive workout regimen and state of wellness.

CHAPTER 6
NORDIC WALKING FOR WEIGHT LOSS

A growing trend in the fitness industry, Nordic walking has garnered interest due to its potential as a weight loss aid. Nordic walking is predicated on the application of walking poles with anatomical features that target the muscles of the upper body in conjunction with those of the lower body. This comprehensive activation of all body parts leads to an increased expenditure of calories in comparison to conventional walking. When developing a Nordic walking regimen for weight loss, it is critical to take into account various elements including intensity, duration, frequency, and progression. Research has demonstrated that the integration of interval training, characterized by alternating high and low walking intensities, can effectively increase caloric expenditure and facilitate weight loss.

A progressive program in which the duration and intensity of Nordic walking sessions are progressively increased can also assist individuals in attaining sustainable long-term weight loss. To maximize weight loss results, it is critical to comprehend the physiological demands of Nordic walking and to customize the program according to the fitness levels of the participants.

<u>Advice on Nutrition for Nordic Walkers:</u>

Although Nordic walking is a highly efficient method for consuming calories and aiding in weight loss, it is crucial to emphasize the utmost importance of nutrition in the pursuit of fitness objectives.

Adequate nutrition not only provides the body with the energy it needs to perform at its peak during Nordic walking sessions but also promotes recuperation and overall health. It is recommended that Nordic walkers adhere to a balanced diet comprising an assortment of nutrient-dense foods, including fruits, vegetables, lean proteins, whole carbohydrates, and healthy fats. Sufficient hydration is critical, particularly when engaging in Nordic walking sessions that are extended in duration or more intense. Given the energy demand linked to this physical activity, participants in Nordic walking ought to be mindful of their caloric consumption, aiming to maintain a marginally negative balance in calories to facilitate weight loss. Nutritional strategies can also differ by individual objectives, such as enhancing physical fitness, losing weight, or gaining muscle. Dietitians and nutritionists can assist Nordic walkers in optimizing the health benefits of their exercise regimen through the modification of their dietary practices.

<u>Achievements and Testimonials:</u>

Attestations and success stories are pivotal in promoting the weight loss benefits of Nordic walking. The following anecdotes present the personal experiences of individuals who effectively accomplished their objectives of weight loss by adhering to a regular Nordic walking regimen. Gaining an understanding of the experiences of others who are undertaking their weight loss journey can inspire and motivate those who are just beginning. Success stories frequently emphasize the profound effects that Nordic walking has on an individual's physical health, mental state, and overall way of life. Additionally, testimonials may illuminate the difficulties individuals encountered and how they surmounted barriers while attempting to lose weight via Nordic walking. These narratives foster a sense of camaraderie and assistance, thereby cultivating a favourable atmosphere for those aspiring to begin or maintain a Nordic walking regimen. By integrating success stories and testimonials into fitness programs, promotional materials, and educational materials, the allure of Nordic walking as a practical and readily available method for attaining weight loss objectives can be significantly augmented.

Engaging both the upper and lower body musculature, Nordic walking has become recognized as an effective method for achieving weight loss. A Nordic walking program that is effective for weight loss requires meticulous consideration of intensity, duration, frequency, and progression, among other elements. The role of nutrition in supporting the demands of Nordic walking is crucial, and to optimize the benefits of their exercise regimen, individuals should employ a well-balanced diet. The endorsement of Nordic walking as a weight loss method is aided by success stories and testimonials, which furnish concrete instances of individuals who have successfully attained their physical fitness objectives by engaging in this activity.

In general, the integration of a meticulously planned Nordic walking regimen, appropriate dietary practices, and the inspiration garnered from triumph tales can galvanize individuals to commence a prosperous metabolic journey via Nordic walking.

CHAPTER 7
INVESTIGATING NORDIC WALKING TRAILS

. Nordic walking, which originated in Finland during the 1930s, has since developed into a well-liked total-body workout involving the use of specialized walking poles. As more individuals participate in this form of physical exercise, the investigation of Nordic walking trails assumes a pivotal role in the overall experience. Urban Nordic walking routes afford participants the chance to effortlessly incorporate this low-impact form of exercise into urban environments. By frequently passing through parks, sidewalks, and cityscapes, these routes enable individuals to integrate physical activity into their everyday schedules.

The incorporation of Nordic walking into urban settings promotes inclusivity and accessibility, accommodating individuals with varying degrees of physical fitness.

Conversely, wilderness exploration and nature trails provide an incongruous yet equally gratifying encounter. Nordic trekkers engage in a profound immersion in the picturesque terrains of nature, traversing forests, mountains, and other scenic features.

Nature trails' undulating topography compels hikers to utilize various muscle groups, thereby augmenting the overall efficacy of the exercise regimen. The aforementioned affinity with the natural world yields psychological advantages, fostering mental health by allowing individuals to inhale pure air and encounter the therapeutic impacts of outdoor settings.

Urban Nordic walking routes are meticulously designed pathways that are constructed entirely within the confines of a city, to accommodate Nordic walkers. The design of these routes facilitates their seamless integration into urban environments, providing individuals desiring a low-impact full-body workout with a convenient and accessible option.

As a rule, these routes traverse a spectrum of topographies, including hilly urban parks and level sidewalks, to guarantee a dynamic and captivating workout encounter. Frequently featuring landmarks and points of interest, urban Nordic walking routes motivate participants to investigate their environment while capitalizing on the advantages of this distinctive mode of physical activity.

Furthermore, the urban infrastructure is intentionally planned to provide Nordic walkers with the necessary facilities, including designated walking lanes, informative signage, and areas for pausing.

In addition to promoting safety, this infrastructure cultivates a sense of community among individuals who are enthusiastic about Nordic walking. In addition to facilitating organized events and group strolls, urban routes serve to enhance the social dimension of this form of physical activity. Fundamentally, urban Nordic walking routes provide a comprehensive and easily accessible method for people to experience the health advantages of Nordic walking amidst the fast-paced environment of the city.

Nature Trails and Wilderness Exploration: In contrast to urban routes, Nordic walking devotees are treated to a more immersive and demanding experience on nature trails and wilderness exploration.

The trails wind through a variety of natural environments, ranging from verdant forests to rugged mountainous regions, thereby offering a scenic backdrop for physical activity.

The nature trail terrain is undulating, necessitating pedestrians to modify their techniques to activate various muscle groups and enhance the cardiovascular component of the exercise.

Nordic walkers may encounter a variety of terrains during wilderness exploration, including rocky paths, dirt pathways, and stream crossings. This diversity not only enhances the overall experience with an element of excitement but also contributes to the comprehensive nature of the exercise routine.

Engaging in wilderness exploration and nature trails provides individuals with the chance to reconnect with the natural world and establish a more profound connection with the environment. Engaging in such immersion can yield significant mental and emotional advantages, including the mitigation of tension and the promotion of a general sense of wellness.

Ensuring Safety and Emergency Readiness: Safety measures and emergency readiness are critical factors in Nordic walking, guaranteeing that participants can partake in this Endeavor with assurance while mitigating potential hazards. In light of the diverse topographies and surroundings encountered during Nordic walking, participants are obligated to strictly adhere to fundamental safety protocols.

This entails donning suitable footwear that offers stability across various terrains, in addition to utilizing Nordic walking poles of superior quality that are specifically engineered to endure the strenuous nature of the activity.

Furthermore, practitioners must be aware of their physical limitations and select trails that correspond with their current levels of fitness. Stretching and warm-up regimens are of the utmost importance to mitigate the risk of injury, particularly when confronted with difficult terrains. Regarding emergency preparedness, Nordic walkers ought to be furnished with indispensable commodities, including communication devices, a first aid kit, and information regarding emergency egress routes. Particularly crucial in remote wilderness environments where immediate access to medical assistance may be scarce is this degree of preparedness.

Educational initiatives and training programs have the potential to significantly influence the dissemination of safety information among devotees of Nordic walking. Workshops that cover emergency response protocols, proper technique, and equipment utilization can enable participants to make informed decisions and engage in the activity responsibly.

By placing a high value on emergency preparedness and safety measures, the Nordic walking community can cultivate an environment that promotes overall wellness, thereby optimizing the physical and mental advantages of this activity while reducing potential hazards.

CHAPTER 8
COMMUNITY AND NORDIC WALKING EVENTS

In addition to becoming a popular physical activity, Nordic Walking has also become a social phenomenon. Active participation in Nordic Walking events and community membership fosters a sense of inclusion and a collective sense of objective among participants. Participating in Nordic Walking groups constitutes a substantial component of this communal Endeavor. These groups frequently comprise individuals from diverse backgrounds and fitness levels, who are brought together by their shared passion for Nordic Walking. Individuals who become members of such organizations are afforded the chance to exchange experiences, gain knowledge from their peers, and cultivate a nurturing atmosphere. Novices can benefit from the advice and equipment recommendations of more experienced walkers in these environments.

Engaging in Nordic Walking competitions enhances the communal dimension of this activity by introducing an additional level of anticipation and difficulty. The level of intensity observed in Nordic Walking competitions varies, encompassing both local and international events. These events function as a medium to exhibit the abilities of accomplished walkers while also fostering the connection of enthusiasts from various social classes. Participating in these competitions may inspire those who are striving to increase their fitness and skill levels.

The presence of competition cultivates a sense of camaraderie among participants, motivating them to surpass their limitations and commemorate the accomplishments of one another. Within the framework of a Nordic Walking competition, the concept of community transcends local organizations and encompasses an expansive network of individuals who are similarly motivated by their ardor for the activity.

Establishing and maintaining a cohesive Nordic Walking community is of paramount importance to foster enduring participation and enhance the general welfare of its members.

This requires fostering an environment that is welcoming to people of all ages and levels of physical endurance. Community-building endeavors may encompass the coordination of social events, seminars, workshops, and seminars that assemble pedestrians beyond the confines of routine sessions. These occasions promote social engagements, enabling attendees to establish significant interpersonal bonds. Moreover, community development transcends in-person exchanges and encompasses digital platforms as well, allowing individuals to maintain connections and participate in dialogues about Nordic Walking. Through the cultivation of a cohesive community, Nordic Walking transcends its physical nature and evolves into a way of life that promotes communal engagement, reciprocal assistance, and a collective dedication to personal growth and wellness.

The involvement of the community and Nordic Walking events is crucial in augmenting the holistic experience of practitioners.

 Nordic walking groups offer members a sense of camaraderie and a forum for the interchange of information; competition participation adds to the fun and cultivates a spirit that is both competitive and encouraging. It is vital to establish a robust Nordic Walking community to foster an environment that is welcoming and inclusive, thereby promoting participants' long-term engagement and general well-being.

CHAPTER 9
CONNECTION OF MIND AND BODY IN NORDIC WALKING

Nordic Walking transcends the mere physical exertion component by integrating a significant focus on the interplay between the mind and body. The practice is founded upon the fundamental principle of mind-body integration. During the Nordic Walking exercise regimen, participants are advised to maintain awareness of their respiration, movements, and overall sensations. Nordic Walking encourages a heightened awareness of body positioning through the harmonious synchronization of upper and lower body movements facilitated by the use of specially designed poles. By intentionally attending to the interplay between the mind and body, one not only amplifies the efficacy of the exercise but also fosters a comprehensive state of wellness.

The mind-body connection exhibited during Nordic Walking may have a positive effect on mental health, according to research.

The walking pattern's rhythmic and repetitive qualities, in conjunction with the arm muscles being engaged via the poles, facilitate the attainment of a meditative state. This attribute of meditation may result in decreased stress and enhanced mental clarity. Research has indicated that participants in mindful Nordic Walking observe mood enhancements and a reduction in symptoms associated with anxiety and depression. By intentionally concentrating on the current moment with each step, one develops a mindful awareness that transcends the duration of the walking session, thereby exerting a positive impact on overall mental resilience.

Moreover, the mental-physical integration observed in Nordic Walking is intricately tied to the notion of proprioception, which pertains to the body's capacity to discern its spatial location. During Nordic Walking, as participants traverse diverse terrains, the interplay between the mind and body generates increased proprioceptive awareness through a feedback cycle. In addition to promoting enhanced balance and coordination, this heightened awareness fosters a more profound connection with the body. Regular practitioners frequently attest to a heightened level of bodily consciousness, resulting in a deeper comprehension of posture and movement patterns.

This enhanced awareness can yield enduring advantages in terms of injury prevention and overall physical wellness.

<u>Meditation on Walking Methods:</u>

Nordic walking incorporates mindful walking techniques as a fundamental component, emphasizing the deliberate and conscientious execution of every step. In contrast to traditional walking, which may emphasize destination attainment, mindful walking in Nordic Walking places greater emphasis on the process rather than the final result. It is recommended that practitioners give careful consideration to the bodily sensations associated with walking, including the foot's contact with the ground, arm swing, and respiratory cadence. Engaging in mindful walking entails developing an attuned awareness of the current moment devoid of evaluation, thereby enabling one to completely engross oneself in the act of walking.

A fundamental component of mindful Nordic walking is the harmonization of the respiratory system with the body's motion. By coordinating their breathing patterns with the swaying motion of their arms and the positioning of the poles, practitioners are instructed. In addition to augmenting the cardiovascular advantages of the activity, this synchronization fosters a state of mindfulness and fluidity.

By deliberately coordinating breath and movement, a rhythmic cadence is produced that promotes relaxation and tension reduction by calming the nervous system.

Furthermore, the practice of mindful walking in Nordic Walking promotes the complete engagement of one's senses. This involves developing an awareness of the visual, auditory, and olfactory stimuli present in the vicinity. Through complete engagement in the sensorial experience of walking, individuals can foster a deeper connection with the natural world and cultivate a sense of stability. Research has shown that the integration of meditative walking techniques into the Nordic Walking regimen can result in enhanced cognitive function and attention. Walking induces a deliberate concentration on the current moment, which amplifies cognitive involvement and yields physical and mental advantages.

Nordic Walking for the Reduction of Stress:

Nordic walking has garnered attention as a potentially beneficial practice for mitigating stress, due to its distinctive amalgamation of physical exertion and mindfulness. In conjunction with the use of poles, the rhythmic and coordinated movements produce an immersive experience that can effectively alleviate tension and its symptoms. Engaging in Nordic Walking induces the release of endorphins, which are endogenous stress relievers and positively impact an individual's overall state of health and wellness.

An important mechanism by which Nordic Walking induces a reduction in tension is its influence on the autonomic nervous system.

 It has been demonstrated that participation in this activity alters the equilibrium between the sympathetic and parasympathetic branches of the autonomic nervous system, resulting in a transition to a state of greater relaxation.

This effect is further enhanced by the incorporation of mindful walking techniques, which induce a meditative and mindful state in opposition to the physiological stress response.

Moreover, Nordic walking affords participants the chance to detach from the pressures of mundane existence and establish a profound connection with the natural world.

The symphony created by the outdoor environment and the synchronized walking patterns provide an opportunity to unwind and seek refuge from the pressures of city life. Existing research has established that stress reduction can be achieved through exposure to nature. Nordic Walking, which prioritizes external engagement, is consistent with this fundamental principle.

Moreover, the stress-relieving benefits of Nordic Walking are further enhanced by its social component. Group Nordic Walking sessions foster a sense of camaraderie and solidarity, enabling participants to exchange personal anecdotes and establish meaningful social bonds. The collective objective and sense of camaraderie can augment the activity's overall beneficial impacts on stress relief. In its entirety, Nordic Walking presents itself as a comprehensive methodology for mitigating stress, attending to the physiological and psychological aspects of this condition.

Stretching and Yoga for Nordic Walkers:

The integration of yoga and stretching exercises into the Nordic Walking regimen contributes a significant aspect to the holistic welfare of participants. Yoga, by its focus on flexibility, equilibrium, and mindfulness, enhances the physical requirements of Nordic Walking, thereby augmenting the overall fitness regimen with a more holistic and integrated approach.

Yoga functions admirably as either a prelude or postlude to Nordic Walking, assisting in the body's recovery or preparing it for the activity. Warming up the muscles and joints with dynamic stretches before Nordic walking can improve flexibility and reduce the risk of injury. By performing these stretches, which can specifically target the hip flexors, quadriceps, and hamstrings, one can ensure that the body is sufficiently primed for the dynamic and rhythmic motions that comprise Nordic Walking.

Post-walk yoga sessions hold equivalent significance as they afford practitioners the chance to relax and partake in static stretches. This facilitates flexibility and prevents muscle rigidity, thereby supporting the recovery process. The addition of yoga to the post-walk regimen may further enhance the relaxation response, thereby complementing the stress-alleviating advantages associated with Nordic Walking.

Stretching exercises that are tailored to Nordic walking specifically target the joints and muscles that are in active motion throughout the activity. This consists of shoulder, arm, and upper back stretches, which target the areas that experience the greatest strain during the pole-assisted movements. Additionally, it is vital to stretch the quadriceps, hip flexors, and calf muscles to prevent rigidity and preserve flexibility.

Additionally, yoga serves to augment the mindfulness component of Nordic Walking. The harmonious integration of attentive walking techniques in Nordic Walking and the contemplative and purposeful essence of yoga facilitates a smooth transition between the two activities. Nordic Walking can benefit from the breath awareness developed through yoga, as it fosters an uninterrupted connection between the breath and the body.

By incorporating yoga and stretching into the Nordic Walking regimen, a comprehensive approach to both physical fitness and mental health is achieved. Through the integration of the dynamic and aerobic components of Nordic Walking with the mindfulness and flexibility of yoga, individuals can attain a synergistic outcome that significantly improves their overall well-being and energy.

CHAPTER 10
NORDIC WALKING AND MENTAL HEALTH

Nordic walking, an exercise regimen incorporating the use of purpose-built poles, has garnered considerable attention due to its manifold health advantages, extending beyond physical fitness and fostering psychological wellness. This essay delves into the cognitive advantages of Nordic Walking, its influence on mental well-being, and how mindfulness is integrated into each stride.

Benefits to the Mind of Nordic Walking

The cognitive advantages of Nordic Walking transcend the activity's physical components. Consistent participation in Nordic walking has been shown to positively influence cognitive functions, including attention, memory, and executive functions, according to research.

The execution of Nordic Walking necessitates intricate motor patterns that demand concentration and coordination, thereby inducing heightened neural activity in brain areas linked to cognitive control. Research has indicated that the cognitive tasks performed during Nordic Walking, which requires the coordination of limb movements, may improve cognitive performance across multiple domains.

Additionally, Nordic walking has been associated with enhanced cognitive acuity and innovation. In addition to engaging upper body musculature, the activity's rhythmic and repetitive characteristics may potentially elicit a meditative state, thereby enhancing mental clarity and concentration. One may find this facet of Nordic Walking to be relevant for individuals who are attempting to improve their cognitive abilities or who are afflicted with neurodegenerative disorders. Therefore, an investigation into the cognitive advantages of Nordic Walking can enhance our overall comprehension of how physical activities influence cognitive processes.

The Benefits of Nordic Walking for Mental Health

Beyond its cognitive advantages, Nordic Walking has garnered recognition for its beneficial impacts on psychological well-being. Participating in consistent physical exercise, such as Nordic Walking, has been linked to the secretion of endorphins, which are endogenous mood enhancers within the body. Nordic Walking, by its rhythmic and full-body characteristics, has the potential to promote stress reduction and mitigate symptoms commonly associated with anxiety and depression. Research has demonstrated that engagement in Nordic Walking programs can result in substantial enhancements in mood and alleviation of tension levels.

Furthermore, Nordic Walking offers a low-impact exercise alternative, thereby ensuring its accessibility to a diverse population, including individuals who are hindered by physical limitations or health conditions. The inclusive nature of Nordic Walking enhances its potential positive effects on mental health by allowing a greater number of individuals to participate without the concern of worsening pre-existing health conditions. The communal nature of Nordic Walking, which is frequently executed in groups, contributes to psychological health by promoting a feeling of support and community.

Integrating Mindfulness into Each Action

The incorporation of mindfulness, which entails being entirely present and attentive in the present moment, into Nordic Walking can be achieved effortlessly. By combining the rhythmic motion of walking with the use of poles, individuals are afforded a singular opportunity to concentrate on the present moment. By performing each step intentionally and mindfully, a connection is established between the body and mind.

Engaging in mindfulness while Nordic walking entails directing one's attention toward bodily sensations, respiration, and immediate surroundings.

Integrating mindfulness into each stride of Nordic Walking may yield significant benefits in terms of mitigating tension and enhancing overall psychological health. Engaging in this activity fosters a state of mindfulness and relaxation, both of which are conducive to a reduction in stress, which can be especially advantageous for those coping with the pressures of contemporary society. Existing research has demonstrated that the integration of mindfulness-based interventions with physical activity, such as Nordic walking, can augment the beneficial impacts on mental well-being.

Nordic walking is recognized not solely as a form of physical exercise, but also as a comprehensive strategy for enhancing mental health. Nordic Walking is a multifaceted activity that offers individuals seeking to improve their physical and mental health numerous advantages, including cognitive benefits, mental health benefits, and the integration of mindfulness into each step. Gaining insight into the dynamic relationship between Nordic Walking and mental well-being presents opportunities for additional scholarly inquiry and the creation of individualized interventions that cater to the needs of various demographic groups.

CHAPTER 11
NUTRITION AND HYDRATION FOR NORDIC WALKERS

Nordic walking, a widely practiced and energetic form of physical activity, necessitates thoughtful deliberation regarding nutrition and hydration to maximize performance and general welfare. The implementation of pre-walk nutrition strategies is critical in guaranteeing that Nordic walkers possess adequate energy levels to endure the strenuous physical demands of their activity. Carbohydrates, being the principal energy source during endurance activities, therefore, assume an essential function in pre-walk nutrition. A slow-release energy source, such as complex carbohydrates (e.g., fruits and whole cereals), should be consumed a few hours before a Nordic walking session to prevent early fatigue and increase endurance.

After carbohydrates, sufficient protein consumption is critical for the maintenance and repair of muscles. Nordic walkers should incorporate lean protein sources into their pre-walk meals, such as poultry, salmon, or plant-based alternatives. Maintaining energy balance is crucial for Nordic walking, as it guarantees consistent energy levels for the duration of the exercise session. Additionally, meal timing should be taken into account; consuming a nutritious meal two to three hours before engaging in physical activity promotes optimal digestion and absorption of nutrients.

The importance of hydration is equivalent when it comes to Nordic walking.

Ensuring adequate fluid balance is critical for optimal performance and general well-being. It is recommended that hydration begin in advance of the walking session, and walkers should strive to consume an adequate amount of water throughout the day. Frequent hydration is advised during Nordic walking, especially during protracted or vigorous sessions, to avert dehydration. Additionally, electrolyte-rich beverages may aid in the replacement of salts lost via perspiration, particularly in warmer climates or during extended physical exertion.

The importance of post-walk recuperation nutrition in the overall nutritional strategy of a Nordic walker is frequently overlooked.

The body necessitates restoration of impaired muscle tissue and replenishment of depleted energy reserves following the conclusion of a session. After engaging in physical activity, consuming a blend of carbohydrates and protein within the initial 30-60 minutes promotes recovery through the facilitation of muscle protein synthesis and the replenishment of glycogen stores. For optimal recovery following a walk, it is advisable to consume nutrient-dense munchies or meals. For instance, a balanced meal comprising lean protein and whole grains or a protein smoothie with fruits can be effective.

The comprehension and application of these nutritional strategies may have a substantial influence on the endurance, recuperation, and performance of Nordic walkers. Maximizing the benefits of this physically taxing activity requires a nutritional strategy that is both well-balanced and appropriately timed.

<u>Maintenance and Selection of Equipment for Nordic Walking:</u>

Due to the unique utilization of walking poles, Nordic walking necessitates meticulous deliberation regarding the selection and upkeep of equipment. The efficacy and safety of Nordic walking are significantly impacted by the selection of poles. The selection of walking poles should be determined by an individual's height and gait.

Poles that are adjustable permit customization, thereby ensuring that each stride is properly aligned and that energy is transferred efficiently. Furthermore, it is advisable to contemplate the ergonomics and security of the harness design and grip to optimize the overall walking experience.

The consistent efficacy and longevity of Nordic walking poles are contingent upon their routine maintenance. Consistent examination of pole components, such as straps, grips, and ends, is essential to detect any indications of deterioration or injury. It is imperative to promptly repair or replace damaged poles to prevent harm and preserve their optimal performance. During strolling sessions, lubricating and cleaning adjustable mechanisms and locking systems ensure their proper operation and prevent complications.

Another essential component to consider when selecting equipment for Nordic trekkers is footwear. Footwear must offer sufficient support, cushioning, and stability. Trail shoes featuring a durable tread pattern are advisable for Nordic walkers who favour off-road excursions. Sizing properly is critical to mitigate potential distress and foot complications. Consistent evaluation of footwear condition, with particular attention to the tread, is imperative to guarantee a stable foothold across diverse terrains.

Nordic walkers who wish to maximize the benefits of their activity must possess a fundamental comprehension of the methods underlying equipment selection and maintenance. Adequately maintained and judiciously chosen equipment not only improves performance but also contributes to the safety and satisfaction of the Nordic walking experience as a whole.

Technique and Biomechanics in Nordic Walking:

Nordic walking, characterized by its distinctive pole-assisted walking technique, incorporates particular biomechanical principles and methodologies that enhance its efficacy as a total-body workout. A comprehensive comprehension of the biomechanics involved in Nordic Walking is essential to attain appropriate form and optimize the activation of diverse muscle groups.

By engaging the upper body, torso, and lower extremities in a coordinated and rhythmic fashion, the poles function as dynamic tools.

A fundamental component of the biomechanics of Nordic Walking is the arm movement. The arm swing, when performed in conjunction with the opposite limb, generates a natural pendulum effect that improves the propulsion and efficiency of every stride.

By introducing resistance and necessitating the active involvement of the shoulders, arms, and abdominal muscles, the poles contribute to this arm swing. In addition to facilitating energy transfer, an appropriate arm motion fosters a rhythmic and balanced gait.

The efficacy of Nordic Walking is intrinsically linked to technique.

Precise timing, the appropriate placement of poles, and the angle of the wrist harnesses are all essential elements that constitute proper technique.

To maintain stability and control, Nordic walkers should position the poles at an angle behind and to the side of the body, engaging the core muscles. Adjusting the wrist straps to provide a secure hold without excessive tension will facilitate the efficient use of the poles.

A fluent and natural Nordic walking gait also requires mastery of the rolling motion of the foot, which extends from heel strike to toe-off. By effectively coordinating arm motion, pole placement, and foot mechanics, an orchestrated and streamlined movement pattern is generated, thereby optimizing the cardiovascular and muscular advantages derived from the exercise.

Individuals must comprehend the biomechanics and technique of Nordic Walking to fully exploit the benefits of this distinctive exercise modality. Achieving proficiency in these principles not only improves performance but also reduces the likelihood of injury, thereby guaranteeing a secure and pleasurable Nordic walking experience.

Aspects of Psychology Regarding Nordic Walking:

In addition to its physical attributes, Nordic Walking encompasses psychological components that substantially enhance its allure and effectiveness as a comprehensive form of exercise.

The interrelation between the psyche and body is crucial to the Nordic Walking experience as a whole. The activity's rhythmic and repetitive characteristics, in conjunction with the utilization of numerous muscle groups, elicit a state of mental relaxation and mindfulness.

Nordic walking is frequently compared to a vigorous form of meditation. In conjunction with the consistent rhythm of pole placement, the repetitive arm and limb movements produce a meditative cadence that facilitates mental clarity and stress reduction.

The contemplative dimension of Nordic Walking has been associated with mood enhancements, reduced anxiety, and improved holistic health.

Moreover, the psychological benefits of Nordic Walking are frequently enhanced by the outdoor environment in which it is conducted. There are numerous mental health benefits associated with nature, including reduced tension and enhanced mood. The synergistic effect produced by the combination of physical activity and exposure to natural surroundings cultivates a favourable psychological environment for individuals who engage in Nordic walking.

Social factors are of equal importance in the realm of psychology as they pertain to Nordic walking. Sessions of Nordic walking in a group offer prospects for interpersonal engagement, encouragement, and solidarity. A sense of affiliation with a community comprising individuals who share similar interests and goals increases both motivation and commitment to the activity. Nordic walking fosters social cohesion and positive reinforcement, thereby contributing to a beneficial psychological effect.

In addition to its physical advantages, Nordic Walking offers psychological benefits that incorporate stress reduction, social connectivity, and mental well-being.

By acknowledging and incorporating these psychological aspects, the overall desirability and viability of Nordic Walking as a holistic exercise program are improved.

CHAPTER 12
CONQUERING OBSTACLES AND OBSTACLES

Popular physical activity Nordic walking provides numerous health benefits; however, similar to any fitness regimen, it is not devoid of obstacles and setbacks. Frequently, participants encounter challenges that demand unwavering resolve and resilience to surmount. An initial obstacle that stands out is the formidable task of mastering the appropriate technique. Utilizing specially designed poles, each step of Nordic walking necessitates a coordinated and rhythmic motion. Inexperienced walkers might find it difficult to coordinate their limb and arm movements, which could result in frustration.

Nevertheless, through appropriate instruction and consistent effort, people can progressively surmount this obstacle and fully benefit from the Endeavor.

Another noteworthy obstacle pertains to the identification of appropriate terrains for Nordic strolling. Nordic walking is more effective than conventional walking on uneven terrain, hills, and trails. Urban environments might not consistently offer optimal conditions for this pursuit, and individuals might face difficulties in identifying suitable locations. Exploration of parks, nature reserves, or Nordic walking trails becomes imperative in this regard, underscoring the significance of infrastructure development and community support in promoting the accessibility of these areas.

<u>Managing Adverse Weather Conditions:</u>

The elements can significantly impede the safety and enjoyment of Nordic walkers due to the difficulties that the weather can present. Abnormally high or low temperatures have the potential to significantly affect the overall experience. Participants are further confronted with the obstacle of ice conditions and slippery surfaces in colder regions.

Sufficient readiness, encompassing suitable outerwear and footwear, is critical to alleviate the hazards linked to inclement weather. Furthermore, it is imperative to comprehend the physiological reactions associated with various temperatures to maximize performance and mitigate the risk of weather-related injuries.

Inadequate weather and precipitation pose additional obstacles, putting the perseverance and commitment of Nordic walkers to the test. Wet surfaces have the potential to impair the traction of walking poles, which may result in accidents or injuries.

Water-resistant equipment utilization, adherence to correct posture, and adaptation of walking techniques are critical strategies that become indispensable under such circumstances. Furthermore, it is critical to consider the psychological dimension of weather-related difficulties; fostering a constructive mentality and placing emphasis on the revitalizing advantages of engaging in outdoor activities can both aid in surmounting such challenges.

<u>Prevention and Recovery from Injuries:</u>

Prevention of injuries is critical for all physical activities, including Nordic walking. It is essential to comprehend the activity's biomechanics to prevent common injuries caused by improper technique or misuse. Participants may develop stress injuries, specifically affecting the knees and ankles, if they neglect to adhere to the appropriate form. Consequently, imparting knowledge regarding proper posture, arm mechanics, and weight distribution is essential for the prevention of injuries. Furthermore, the integration of suitable warm-up and cool-down exercises into the Nordic walking regimen has the potential to augment flexibility and mitigate the likelihood of strains or sprains.

It is critical to adopt a comprehensive approach to recovery in the unfortunate circumstance of an injury. Nordic walking devotees might find it necessary to make temporary adjustments to their exercise regimen or consult with sports medicine specialists or physiotherapists for assistance.

Rehabilitation exercises that target flexibility improvement and strength training in the afflicted areas have the potential to accelerate the recovery process. Moreover, cultivating a communal atmosphere within the realm of Nordic walking can furnish individuals with the necessary encouragement and drive required to persevere through the arduous phases of recuperating from injuries.

Maintaining Motivation While Nordic Walking:

Ensuring sustained motivation during the Nordic walking voyage is a pivotal determinant of adherence to this exercise modality over the long term. The gradual reduction in initial enthusiasm that accompanies the commencement of a fitness regimen necessitates the investigation of methods that maintain involvement. Goal setting is an efficacious motivational mechanism that enables individuals to define unambiguous objectives and significant milestones. Establishing attainable and quantifiable objectives, whether to surpass difficult terrains, increase distance, or pace, instills a sense of accomplishment and direction.

Ensuring variety in the Nordic walking regimen is an additional critical element in mitigating monotony and maintaining optimal levels of motivation. Incorporating interval training, introducing novel terrains, or investigating additional trails can all contribute to the overall excitement derived from an activity. Moreover, engagement in Nordic walking competitions or membership in clubs cultivates a feeling of communal belonging and companionship, thereby augmenting the overall experience. Social interactions within the Nordic walking community can serve as a source of motivation, providing encouragement and accountability.

Nordic walking, while laden with challenges and setbacks, offers a multifaceted journey filled with physical, mental, and social benefits. Overcoming initial hurdles, adapting to various weather conditions, prioritizing injury prevention, and maintaining motivation are integral aspects of a successful Nordic walking experience. As individuals delve into this unique form of exercise, a comprehensive understanding of these concepts can pave the way for a fulfilling and enduring engagement with Nordic walking.

CHAPTER 13
FUTURE TRENDS IN NORDIC WALKING

<u>Technological Advances in Nordic Walking Gear:</u>

Nordic walking has evolved significantly over the years, and one of the key aspects shaping its future is technological advancements in gear. Traditionally, Nordic walking involved the use of specially designed poles to engage the upper body in the exercise. However, with the integration of technology, the gear used in Nordic walking is transforming. Smart poles equipped with sensors and connectivity features are becoming increasingly popular. These smart poles can track various metrics such as stride length, pole angle, and heart rate, providing walkers with real-time feedback on their performance. Additionally, advanced materials and manufacturing techniques are being employed to create lightweight yet durable poles, enhancing the overall user experience. As technology continues to advance, we can expect further innovations in Nordic walking gear, with the integration of features such as GPS tracking, augmented reality displays, and smart coaching systems.

Emerging Nordic Walking Disciplines:

The world of Nordic walking is expanding beyond its traditional form, and emerging disciplines are contributing to the diversity of this activity. While classic Nordic walking involves brisk walking with the aid of specially designed poles, new disciplines are incorporating different elements to cater to a wider audience. One such emerging discipline is Nordic trail walking, which takes the activity off paved surfaces and onto hiking trails.

This variation adds an element of adventure and challenges participants with uneven terrains, providing a more immersive experience in nature. Another noteworthy development is urban Nordic walking, where individuals engage in the activity within city environments. This adaptation considers the constraints of urban spaces and provides a convenient option for those who may not have access to nature trails. These emerging disciplines not only enhance the versatility of Nordic walking but also cater to different preferences and fitness levels, making it more inclusive and appealing to a broader demographic.

<u>Research and Innovations in the Nordic Walking Community:</u>

The Nordic walking community is actively engaged in research and innovations aimed at further understanding the physiological and psychological benefits of this activity.

Scientific studies are being conducted to explore the impact of Nordic walking on cardiovascular health, muscle strength, and overall well-being. Researchers are using advanced technologies such as motion capture systems and physiological monitoring devices to gather precise data on the biomechanics of Nordic walking. This research is instrumental in refining the techniques and guidelines for practitioners, ensuring optimal health outcomes. Innovations in training methodologies, including virtual reality-enhanced programs and interactive apps, are being developed to make Nordic walking more accessible and enjoyable. Furthermore, there is a growing emphasis on the mental health benefits of Nordic walking, with studies exploring its effects on stress reduction, mood enhancement, and cognitive function.

As the Nordic walking community continues to invest in research and innovations, we can anticipate a deeper understanding of the holistic benefits of this activity, fostering its integration into mainstream health and wellness practices.

the future trends in Nordic walking encompass a range of developments that are poised to shape the trajectory of this popular physical activity. Technological advances in gear, including the integration of smart poles and innovative materials, are enhancing the overall experience for participants.

Emerging disciplines, such as Nordic trail walking and urban Nordic walking, are expanding the reach of Nordic walking, making it more adaptable to diverse environments.

The ongoing research and innovations within the Nordic walking community are contributing to a deeper understanding of its physiological and psychological benefits, paving the way for optimized training methodologies and increased awareness of its holistic advantages. As we look ahead, the evolution of Nordic walking holds promise for a more dynamic, inclusive, and scientifically supported activity in the realm of health and fitness.

CHAPTER 14
ENVIRONMENTAL CONSCIOUSNESS IN NORDIC WALKING

Nordic Walking, a popular fitness activity, has garnered attention not only for its health benefits but also for its environmental consciousness. Participants in Nordic Walking are often inclined towards eco-friendly practices, recognizing the importance of preserving the natural environment while engaging in physical activity. One key aspect of environmental consciousness in Nordic Walking is the choice of equipment. Nordic Walking poles are typically made from lightweight and sustainable materials, reflecting a commitment to reducing the environmental impact of the gear used in the activity.

Furthermore, Nordic Walkers often prioritize walking in natural settings, such as parks, trails, and forested areas. This preference not only enhances the overall experience of Nordic Walking but also aligns with the ethos of environmental sustainability. The act of exercising amidst nature fosters a connection between individuals and their surroundings, instilling a sense of responsibility for the environment. Participants tend to be more aware of the ecosystems they traverse, leading to a greater likelihood of adopting eco-friendly habits beyond their Nordic Walking sessions.

The concept of environmental consciousness in Nordic Walking extends to the disposal of equipment and waste. Nordic Walkers are encouraged to dispose of their gear responsibly, either through recycling programs or other environmentally friendly methods. Additionally, the promotion of a "leave no trace" ethos is common in Nordic Walking communities, emphasizing the importance of minimizing human impact on natural habitats. This conscientious approach to waste management contributes to the overall eco-friendly nature of Nordic Walking.

14.1 Eco-Friendly Practices for Nordic Walkers:

Eco-friendly practices in Nordic Walking encompass a range of behaviours and choices that collectively contribute to minimizing the environmental footprint of the activity. One prominent aspect is the use of sustainable materials in the manufacturing of Nordic Walking equipment. The Nordic Walking poles, in particular, are designed with materials that prioritize durability and low environmental impact. This may include the use of recycled materials or those derived from renewable resources.

In addition to sustainable materials, Nordic Walkers often engage in practices that reduce energy consumption during the production and distribution of equipment. Some individuals opt for locally sourced gear to minimize transportation-related emissions, while others may choose brands that actively engage in carbon offset programs. These considerations highlight a growing awareness within the Nordic Walking community regarding the interconnectedness of their activity with broader environmental concerns.

Another key eco-friendly practice is the conscious choice of walking routes. Nordic Walkers are encouraged to select paths that promote biodiversity and natural preservation. Avoiding sensitive habitats and respecting wildlife is integral to these practices. Many Nordic Walking groups collaborate with environmental organizations to develop guidelines for responsible trail use, ensuring that participants are well-informed about the impact of their chosen routes on local ecosystems.

14.2 Conservation Initiatives and Nordic Walking:

Conservation initiatives within the Nordic Walking community demonstrate a commitment to preserving natural environments and promoting sustainability beyond individual practices. These initiatives often involve collaboration between Nordic Walking organizations, environmental groups, and local authorities. One common strategy is the establishment and maintenance of dedicated Nordic Walking trails within protected areas. These trails are carefully designed to minimize disruption to ecosystems while providing participants with a scenic and enjoyable experience.

Furthermore, Nordic Walking events and competitions frequently align themselves with conservation causes. Fundraising efforts may be directed toward environmental projects, such as reforestation, wildlife protection, or the restoration of natural habitats. This not only enhances the positive impact of Nordic Walking on the environment but also fosters a sense of community and shared responsibility among participants.

Conservation-focused education plays a crucial role in Nordic Walking initiatives. Participants are often informed about the ecological significance of the areas they traverse, learning about local flora and fauna, and understanding the importance of biodiversity. This knowledge empowers Nordic Walkers to become advocates for conservation, encouraging them to spread awareness and actively contribute to the protection of natural resources.

the concepts of environmental consciousness, eco-friendly practices, and conservation initiatives are integral components of the Nordic Walking experience. As the popularity of this activity continues to grow, participants, organizers, and manufacturers need to prioritize sustainability and environmental responsibility. Through these efforts, Nordic Walking can not only contribute to individual health and well-being but also serve as a model for harmonious coexistence between recreational activities and the natural world.

Nordic Walking, with its origins deeply rooted in Finland as a summer training method for cross-country skiers, has evolved into a versatile exercise modality suitable for individuals across various age groups and fitness levels. In particular, its application for special populations showcases the adaptability and inclusive nature of this physical activity.

15.1 Nordic Walking for Children and Teens

Introducing Nordic Walking to children and teens not only addresses the increasing sedentary lifestyle but also fosters a lifelong commitment to physical activity. The biomechanical aspect of Nordic Walking, incorporating the use of poles, enhances the engagement of upper body muscles, promoting balanced muscle development. It further instills appropriate posture and gait patterns, which are crucial during the formative years. The rhythmic and dynamic nature of Nordic Walking can make it more appealing to younger individuals compared to conventional walking or running, contributing to sustained interest and participation. Additionally, as a low-impact exercise, Nordic Walking reduces the risk of injuries, making it a safe option for developing musculoskeletal systems. Research exploring the cognitive benefits of Nordic Walking for children and teens, such as enhanced attention span and academic performance, highlights its potential as a holistic approach to youth development.

15.2 Nordic Walking for Individuals with Disabilities

Nordic Walking emerges as an inclusive exercise modality for individuals with disabilities, demonstrating its adaptability to diverse physical conditions. The use of poles provides stability, aiding individuals with equilibrium issues or mobility impairments.

For those with upper body strength limitations, the poles distribute the effort, allowing for a more balanced engagement of musculature. Moreover, the rhythmic nature of Nordic Walking can contribute to the development of coordination and motor skills, making it a valuable component in rehabilitation programs for individuals with neurological disorders or injuries. Research in this domain examines the impact of Nordic Walking on specific disabilities, such as Parkinson's disease or spinal cord injuries, underlining the potential for enhancing functional capacity and quality of life. Tailoring Nordic Walking programs to the unique requirements of individuals with disabilities requires a multidisciplinary approach, involving physiotherapists, adaptive physical education specialists, and rehabilitation professionals to ensure safety and efficacy.

15.3 Incorporating Nordic Walking into Rehabilitation Programs

In the domain of rehabilitation, Nordic Walking emerges as a holistic and adaptable intervention that complements traditional approaches. Its low-impact nature, combined with the engagement of both upper and lower body musculature, makes it a suitable activity for individuals recovering from various injuries or surgeries. Incorporating Nordic Walking into rehabilitation programs offers a transitional step between more passive interventions and higher-impact activities, facilitating a progressive progression toward full functional recovery.

The use of poles provides added support, aiding individuals in maintaining balance and reducing the burden on injured joints.

The incorporation of Nordic Walking into rehabilitation regimens for conditions such as knee osteoarthritis or recovery from cardiac surgery is substantiated by research.

Such regimens exhibit favourable results regarding enhanced cardiovascular fitness, joint functionality, and general welfare. Rehabilitation professionals, physiotherapists, and Nordic Walking instructors must work in tandem to customize programs according to the specific requirements of each individual, track progress, and guarantee the secure and efficient integration of this activity into rehabilitation protocols.

The adaptability of Nordic Walking is evident in its utilization with special populations. Nordic Walking is an adaptable and valuable tool that incorporates various demographic groups to promote health and well-being. It does so by involving children and teenagers in a dynamic and enjoyable form of exercise, offering an inclusive option for individuals with disabilities, and seamlessly integrating into rehabilitation programs. The ongoing investigation into the advantages of Nordic Walking for special populations emphasizes the necessity for ongoing research, professional collaboration, and the creation of individualized programs to optimize the beneficial effects of Nordic Walking in these particular settings.

CHAPTER 16
BEYOND FITNESS: NORDIC WALKING AS A LIFESTYLE

Nordic walking, which originated as an alternative summer training activity for cross-country skiers in Finland during the 1930s, is a full-body exercise that has since developed into a multifaceted pursuit that transcends mundane physical fitness. Nordic walking is increasingly being incorporated into everyday life, and enthusiasts are adopting it not only as a form of physical exercise but also as a holistic approach to living. The transition from a basic exercise regimen to a holistic lifestyle entails the integration of Nordic walking into numerous facets of everyday schedules.

Incorporating Nordic Walking into Routine Activities

The notion of incorporating Nordic walking into one's daily routine entails the seamless integration of this form of physical activity into customary duties. In contrast to conventional exercise regimens that consist of designated periods, Nordic walking enables people to incorporate physical activity into their day-to-day activities. This integration accomplishes more than mere fitness objectives; it cultivates a mentality in which engaging in physical activity becomes an intrinsic component of one's daily existence. The notion that Nordic walking can be integrated into routine activities such as commuting, strolling the dog, or socializing with friends is the foundation of this concept.

The objective is to convert physical activity from a designated activity to an ongoing, pervasive practice that enhances well-being as a whole.

The incorporation of Nordic walking into one's daily existence transcends the physical domain and encompasses mental and emotional dimensions as well. As individuals consistently participate in this activity, it transforms into a meditative practice that fosters mindfulness and alleviates tension. The outdoor environment combined with the rhythmic motion of Nordic walking fosters an environment that is conducive to mental relaxation and contemplation. Nordic walking is distinguished from other forms of exercise by its incorporation of mental and physical health benefits; it is a lifestyle choice that advocates for a holistic approach to health.

Exploration and Travel Using Nordic Walking

Nordic strolling, which originates in the Scandinavian countries, has organically evolved into a pastime associated with nature exploration and travel. The notion of traveling and discovering through Nordic walking transcends traditional modes of tourism. Travel is not merely a respite for enthusiasts; it also provides them with the chance to partake in their preferred physical activity in a variety of picturesque settings. Nordic walking serves as a means of exploration, facilitating individuals to establish a connection with the natural world and actively and fully engage with unfamiliar environments.

This notion is intricately linked with the concept of adventure tourism, in which enthusiasts of Nordic walking endeavor to merge their enthusiasm for traversing diverse landscapes. Nature reserves, parks, and trails transform from mere tourist attractions into vibrant spaces that encourage active engagement.

By integrating Nordic walking into travel arrangements, individuals can gain a distinctive perspective that surpasses that of conventional tourist pursuits. The integration of exploration and physical activity in this comprehensive travel approach elevates the overall travel experience and aids in the rise in popularity of Nordic walking as a lifestyle preference.

Nordic Walking Practices That Promote Long-Term Health

The maintenance and sustainability of Nordic walking as a way of life are contingent upon the development of routines that foster enduring health. This notion transcends the immediate advantages of engaging in physical activity and explores the wider domains of well-being, environmental awareness, and societal participation. Sustainable Nordic walking habits comprise a multitude of elements, such as the activity's ecological ramifications, the interpersonal bonds formed throughout collective walks, and the continuous dedication to individual welfare.

From an ecological standpoint, the practice of sustainable Nordic walking entails a diligent

Endeavor to reduce the ecological impact linked to this activity. The promotion of responsible outdoor conduct, adherence to the Leave No Trace principles, and the selection of trails and itineraries that prioritize nature conservation all contribute to the sustainability of Nordic walking as an environmentally conscious way of life. By embracing the natural environment, devotees not only have a backdrop for exercise but also a collective obligation to safeguard and preserve the landscapes they traverse.

Social interaction constitutes an additional pivotal element of sustainable Nordic walking practices. Community events and group treks cultivate a feeling of inclusion and companionship among those who partake. The social dimension of the activity transcends mere physical exertion, fostering a network of support that improves one's mental and emotional health. The sustainability of Nordic walking as a lifestyle choice can be attributed to the communal nature of this approach, whereby the social connections forged during walks serve as an incentive for participants to maintain their dedication to the activity.

In addition, an ongoing dedication to personal health is a component of sustainable Nordic walking practices that promote long-term well-being. This encompasses consistent health examinations, appropriate warm-up and cool-down protocols, and the integration of diverse exercise routines to target various facets of physical fitness. The commitment to comprehensive well-being guarantees that Nordic walking maintains its viability across various life stages, accommodating the evolving capabilities and requirements of participants.

TO CONCLUDE

Nordic walking has transformed its initial purpose as a physical activity to become an all-encompassing way of life. The incorporation of Nordic walking into one's daily routine represents a transition from a structured exercise regimen to a continuous, all-encompassing activity that enhances general health. This lifestyle decision transcends mere physical fitness by integrating mental and emotional dimensions, thereby converting Nordic walking into an activity that promotes meditation and alleviates tension.

The correlation between Nordic walking and travel underscores the multipurpose nature of the activity, as ardent practitioners traverse a variety of topographical regions while integrating physical exertion into their expeditions. This not only amplifies the travel experience but also exemplifies the dynamic and immersive nature of Nordic walking as a means of engaging with the world.

The sustainable Nordic walking practices serve to emphasize the enduring feasibility of this particular way of life. Through the promotion of social connections, the cultivation of holistic health, and the contemplation of environmental consequences, devotees uphold the sustainability and ecological consciousness of Nordic walking. Nordic walking is a sustainable lifestyle choice that transcends fad status by integrating social interaction, environmental consciousness, and physical exercise—all of which contribute to your overall well-being.

Fundamentally, comprehending Nordic walking necessitates acknowledging that it transcends a collection of physical movements and instead represents a philosophical framework that harmoniously amalgamates into diverse aspects of existence. Nordic walking embraces a comprehensive approach to a gratifying and health-conscious way of life, whether it involves integrating into daily routines, enriching travel experiences, or promoting sustainable habits.